Table of Co

Introduction

- Setting the Stage for Mindfulness in a Hectic World
- The Importance of Mindfulness for Busy Professionals
- What to Expect from This Ebook

Chapter 1: Understanding Mindfulness

- Definition and Essence of Mindfulness
- The Roots of Mindfulness: A Brief History
- Mindfulness in Today's Fast-Paced World

Chapter 2: The Mindful Mindset for Professionals

- The Unique Challenges of Busy Professionals
- The Impact of Stress on Performance and Well-being
- The Mindful Professional Advantage

Chapter 3: Embracing Mindfulness: Getting Started

- Preparing Yourself for Mindfulness
- The Mindfulness Mindset
- Creating Your Mindful Space

Chapter 4: Quick Mindfulness Practices for Busy Schedules

- Introduction to "Mindful Moments"
- Mindful Breathing: A Foundation for Presence

- Mindful Mini-Meditations: Finding Stillness in Seconds
- Integrating Mindful Moments into Your Day

Chapter 5: Mindfulness for Stress Reduction

- Stress: The Silent Productivity Killer
- The Science of Mindfulness and Stress Reduction
- Mindfulness-Based Stress Reduction Techniques

Chapter 6: Mindful Communication: Building Better Relationships

- The Power of Mindful Communication
- Mindful Listening: A Gift to Others and Yourself
- Mindful Communication at Work and Home

Chapter 7: Building Resilience Through Mindfulness

- The Role of Mindfulness in Building Resilience
- Strategies for Bouncing Back from Setbacks
- Cultivating a Positive Mindset

Chapter 8: Mindful Tech Use in a Digital World

- The Digital Age Dilemma
- Mindful Tech Practices for Greater Productivity
- Reclaiming Your Time and Attention

Chapter 9: Real-Life Success Stories

- Stories of Transformation: Real Professionals, Real Results
- How Mindfulness Changed Their Careers and Lives

Chapter 10: Creating Your Mindful Lifestyle

- Summarizing the Journey So Far
- Your Mindful Lifestyle Plan: Step-by-Step
- Mindfulness as a Lifelong Companion

Conclusion

- The Power of Mindfulness: A Lasting Legacy
- Embarking on Your Mindfulness Journey
- Thank You for Choosing "On-the-Go Mindfulness"

Additional Resources

- Recommended Books, Websites, and Apps

About the Author

- Author Bio and Contact Information

Endnotes

- Citations and References

Introduction

In an ever-accelerating world, where the pace of life seems to quicken with each passing day, finding moments of respite can feel like an impossible feat. We wake up to a barrage of emails, rush from one obligation to another, and seldom find time to pause and reflect. Yet, in the midst of this relentless whirlwind, there exists a timeless practice—a beacon of serenity—that has never been more relevant. It's called mindfulness, and it holds the power to transform the way we perceive and engage with our bustling world.

Welcome to the realm of mindfulness—a practice that offers an oasis of calm in the desert of busyness. In this introductory section, we'll set the stage for mindfulness, exploring why it has emerged as a vital tool for individuals navigating the demands of modern life. We'll peel back the layers of this age-old practice, revealing its key concepts and the myriad benefits it brings. As we embark on this journey, prepare to discover how mindfulness can be your compass in a hectic world, guiding you toward greater clarity, presence, and well-being.

The Modern Dilemma: A Hectic World

To understand the profound significance of mindfulness in today's world, we must first acknowledge the unique challenges and complexities we face. Picture your typical day—a relentless parade of meetings, emails, deadlines, and responsibilities. The digital age has ushered in an era of constant connectivity, where smartphones tether us to work, social media, and a never-ending stream of information. We are inundated with demands on our time, attention, and energy, often leaving us feeling stretched thin and exhausted.

This is the paradox of our age—unprecedented connectivity juxtaposed with a pervasive sense of disconnection. We're always plugged in, yet seldom truly present. Amid the cacophony of notifications and multitasking, the ability to focus, to immerse ourselves in a single task, and to savor the present moment has become a rare and precious skill.

The consequences of this hectic lifestyle are far-reaching. Stress levels are on the rise, affecting not only our mental and emotional well-being but also our physical health. Research shows that chronic stress is linked to a myriad of health problems, from cardiovascular issues to compromised immune function. In the workplace, stress can lead to burnout, decreased productivity, and strained relationships.

The Power of Mindfulness: A Timeless Solution

In the face of this modern dilemma, mindfulness emerges as a time-tested remedy—a practice that has been cultivated and refined for millennia. At its essence, mindfulness is about presence. It's about paying full and non-judgmental attention to the present moment. This seemingly simple act of presence carries profound implications for our lives.

Mindfulness invites us to step off the relentless treadmill of busyness and find sanctuary in the now. It encourages us to let go of the constant mental chatter, the perpetual planning, and the relentless self-criticism. Instead, it invites us to meet each moment with openness and curiosity, to see the world afresh, and to embrace life's experiences—both pleasant and challenging—with equanimity.

The roots of mindfulness trace back to ancient contemplative traditions, particularly within Buddhism. However, in recent decades, mindfulness has transcended its spiritual origins to become a secular and evidence-based practice. Researchers and psychologists have extensively studied its effects, unveiling a treasure trove of benefits for individuals from all walks of life.

The Importance of Mindfulness for Busy Professionals

In the fast-paced world of modern professionals, the importance of mindfulness cannot be overstated. It's not merely a trendy practice; it's a lifeline—a means to navigate the tumultuous waters of work, responsibilities, and the ever-increasing demands of a connected age.

The Unique Challenges of the Modern Professional

In the bustling landscape of the contemporary professional, each day is a whirlwind of activity, akin to a tightly choreographed dance. Meetings, emails, deadlines, presentations—the calendar is an intricate mosaic of obligations, often resembling a juggler's act, attempting to keep countless balls in the air simultaneously. The relentless pace of the professional world rarely allows for respite. And while the digital age has brought unprecedented convenience, it has also tethered us to a constant stream of information, notifications, and distractions. The boundaries between work and personal life have blurred, making it increasingly challenging to disconnect and find moments of reprieve.

Amidst this unceasing rush, it's easy to lose sight of the importance of well-being. Stress becomes a constant companion, lurking in the background, and often, we're not even aware of its presence until it manifests in physical symptoms, emotional exhaustion, or burnout. The pressures of the professional arena can take a toll on mental health, strain relationships, and hinder overall performance.

The Perils of Stress and Overwhelm

Stress is not merely an inconvenience; it's a significant threat to physical and mental health. Chronic stress has been linked to a range of ailments, from heart disease and high blood pressure to depression and anxiety disorders. For professionals, the pressures of the workplace can serve as a breeding ground for stress and its detrimental effects.

Overwhelm is another common experience for busy professionals. The constant influx of information, decision-making, and multitasking can lead to cognitive overload. You might find yourself in a state of "analysis paralysis," where the sheer volume of tasks and choices paralyzes your ability to make decisions effectively.

Mindfulness as an Antidote

It's in this landscape of stress, overwhelm, and perpetual motion that mindfulness emerges as a powerful antidote. Mindfulness is not an escape from the challenges of the professional world; it's a means to navigate them more skillfully.

Mindfulness invites you to step off the treadmill of busyness, even if just for a moment. It encourages you to pause and observe your thoughts, emotions, and physical sensations without judgment. In doing so, it offers a respite from the ceaseless mental chatter and the unrelenting pace of modern life.

The Mindful Professional Advantage

Beyond stress reduction, mindfulness offers a host of benefits that are particularly advantageous for professionals. It enhances emotional intelligence, fostering greater self-awareness and improved interpersonal relationships. By cultivating a non-judgmental awareness of thoughts and emotions, mindfulness equips you with the tools to navigate complex workplace dynamics with composure and clarity.

Mindfulness also sharpens your focus—a precious skill in an age of distractions. It teaches you to bring your full attention to the task at hand, whether it's preparing a presentation, leading a team meeting, or engaging in a crucial conversation with a colleague or client. In the midst of information overload, mindfulness allows you to sift through the noise and discern what truly matters.

Additionally, mindfulness enhances creativity. When you quiet the mind and let go of the constant mental chatter, you create space for innovative ideas to surface. Professionals who practice mindfulness often find themselves approaching challenges with fresh perspectives, generating novel solutions, and thinking "outside the box."

But perhaps the most profound gift of mindfulness is its ability to infuse each moment with intention and meaning. In an era defined by constant distractions, the practice of mindfulness invites you to savor the richness of the present moment. It allows you to fully engage with life's experiences, whether it's relishing a well-prepared meal, appreciating the laughter of a loved one, or finding joy in a moment of stillness.

The Mindfulness Revolution

The recognition of mindfulness's importance in the professional world has led to a mindfulness revolution. It's not confined to meditation retreats or yoga studios—it's happening in boardrooms, classrooms, and office cubicles. Major corporations, from Google to General Mills, have introduced mindfulness programs for employees, recognizing the positive impact on well-being and productivity. Universities offer mindfulness courses, and even healthcare providers are incorporating mindfulness-based interventions into mental health treatment.

Closing Thoughts

In this exploration of the importance of mindfulness for busy professionals, we've uncovered the unique challenges of the modern professional landscape—the relentless pace, the ever-present stress, and the constant demands on your attention. We've highlighted the perils of stress and overwhelm, emphasizing their impact on both mental and physical well-being.

In response to these challenges, we've introduced mindfulness as a potent antidote—a practice that empowers you to navigate the professional world with greater clarity, resilience, and a profound sense of well-being. We've discussed the advantages of mindfulness for professionals, from enhanced emotional intelligence and improved focus to heightened creativity and a deeper connection with the present moment.

As we proceed through the pages of this ebook, we'll delve deeper into the practical strategies and techniques that allow you to infuse mindfulness into your daily life as a busy professional. We'll explore how to apply mindfulness in the workplace, during your commute, and even in those brief moments of respite during the day. We'll share real-life stories of professionals who have harnessed the power of mindfulness to transform their careers and lives.

Are you ready to embrace mindfulness as your ally in the professional arena? Let's continue our journey into "On-the-Go Mindfulness," where the path to greater clarity, presence, and well-being awaits you.

What to Expect: Navigating "On-the-Go Mindfulness"

As we journey through the pages of this ebook, we'll explore how mindfulness can be your steadfast companion amid the chaos of your professional life. You'll learn not only the principles of mindfulness but also the practical strategies that allow you to infuse mindfulness into your daily routine. We'll introduce the concept of "mindful moments"—short yet powerful exercises that can be seamlessly integrated into your day, whether you're in a meeting, commuting, or simply taking a break.

We'll delve into the science behind mindfulness, demystifying its effects on your brain and well-being. We'll share real-life success stories of busy professionals who have harnessed the power of mindfulness to transform their careers and lives. Most importantly, we'll provide you with actionable steps and guidance to embark on your own mindfulness journey—a journey that promises greater clarity, focus, and a profound sense of well-being.

Are you ready to embrace mindfulness as your compass in a hectic world? Let's begin our exploration of "On-the-Go Mindfulness," where the serenity of the present moment awaits you.

CHAPTER-1

UNDERSTANDING MINDFULNESS

A. Definition and Essence of Mindfulness

At its heart, mindfulness is a profound state of being that transcends the ordinary busyness of our lives. It's a timeless practice with roots that stretch deep into the traditions of contemplative wisdom, yet it's a practice that has never been more relevant than in the fast-paced, hyper-connected world of today's busy professionals. In this section, we'll delve into the very essence of mindfulness, providing you with a clear and comprehensive definition while uncovering the fundamental principles that underpin this transformative practice.

Understanding Mindfulness: A Simple Yet Profound Concept

Mindfulness is often described as the art of being present—fully and non-judgmentally—in the moment. It's about paying attention to your thoughts, emotions, and sensations with a sense of curiosity and acceptance. At its core, mindfulness is deceptively simple, but its impact is profound. Let's break down this definition to understand its essence.

Presence: Mindfulness invites you to show up for your life. It encourages you to engage with each moment, whether it's a mundane task, a challenging situation, or a moment of joy, with your full attention. It's the opposite of going through life on autopilot, where you're physically present but mentally absent.

Non-judgmental: Mindfulness asks you to suspend judgment and criticism. It's about observing your experiences with an open and compassionate heart, without labeling them as good or bad. This non-judgmental stance creates space for self-acceptance and self-compassion.

Thoughts, Emotions, and Sensations: Mindfulness directs your awareness inward. You become the observer of your own inner world. This involves paying attention to your thoughts, the ever-flowing stream of consciousness; your emotions, the ever-shifting landscape of feelings; and your bodily sensations, the physical expressions of your inner state.

Curiosity and Acceptance: Mindfulness invites you to approach your experiences with curiosity, as if you're exploring a new and unfamiliar landscape. It encourages you to meet whatever arises with acceptance, acknowledging that this is the present moment as it is.

The Essence of Mindfulness Practice

Beyond this definition, the essence of mindfulness lies in the cultivation of specific qualities of mind and heart. These qualities are the pillars upon which mindfulness rests, and they shape the way we relate to ourselves, others, and the world around us.

Awareness: Mindfulness begins with awareness. It's the ability to notice what's happening in the present moment without trying to change it. This awareness encompasses your internal experiences (thoughts, emotions, sensations) and your external environment. It's like turning on the light in a dark room, allowing you to see things as they are.

Attention: In the modern world, our attention is constantly fragmented, pulled in a thousand directions. Mindfulness involves training your attention to focus on one thing at a time. This concentrated attention is like a spotlight that illuminates the present moment, helping you see details and nuances you might have otherwise missed.

Equanimity: Equanimity is the quality of remaining calm and balanced, regardless of the circumstances. It's about not being overly reactive or attached to the pleasant or unpleasant experiences that arise. Equanimity allows you to respond to life's challenges with grace and resilience.

Non-reactivity: Mindfulness invites you to respond, not react. It's the ability to pause and choose your response consciously, rather than being driven by automatic reactions. Non-reactivity gives you the freedom to act from a place of wisdom and intention.

Compassion: Mindfulness is not a cold, detached observation of your experiences. It's infused with compassion—compassion for yourself and for others. This compassionate attitude fosters self-acceptance, self-kindness, and empathy for the struggles and suffering of others.

The Paradox of Mindfulness: Simplicity in Complexity

In its essence, mindfulness is simple—being present, non-judgmental, and aware. Yet, it's also deceptively complex. The practice of mindfulness requires commitment and effort. It asks us to unlearn habits of mind that have been deeply ingrained and to cultivate new ways of being.

The paradox of mindfulness is that while it's a practice of simplicity, it has the power to transform the complexity of our lives. It allows us to step out of the constant cycle of doing and into the realm of being. It reveals the richness and depth that exist in the present moment, which we often overlook in our pursuit of the next goal, the next deadline, or the next distraction.

In the pages that follow, we'll guide you through the practice of mindfulness. We'll explore various techniques and exercises that will help you cultivate the qualities of awareness, attention, equanimity, non-reactivity, and compassion. We'll equip you with the tools to integrate mindfulness into your busy professional life, helping you access its transformative power and reap its countless benefits.

Are you ready to embark on this journey of mindfulness, to explore its simplicity, and to unlock its complexity? The path is before you, and the adventure awaits.

B. The Roots of Mindfulness: A Brief History

To understand the origins of mindfulness, we must embark on a journey through time—a journey that takes us to the heart of ancient wisdom and the evolution of a practice that has endured for millennia. In this section, we'll trace the roots of mindfulness, exploring its rich history and the traditions from which it emerged.

Ancient Beginnings: The Origins of Mindfulness

The story of mindfulness begins in the cradle of ancient Eastern wisdom, in the fertile lands of India. It's a story that predates the digital age, the industrial revolution, and even the founding of great empires. The seeds of mindfulness were sown in a culture that valued inner exploration, contemplation, and the search for profound truths.

Early Vedic Traditions: The earliest glimpses of mindfulness can be found in the Vedic traditions of ancient India, which date back over 3,000 years. The Vedas, a collection of sacred texts, contained hymns and rituals that encouraged introspection and meditation. These practices laid the groundwork for the development of mindfulness.

The Buddha's Enlightenment: The true birth of mindfulness, as we understand it today, is often attributed to Siddhartha Gautama, who later became known as the Buddha. In the 5th century BCE, the Buddha embarked on a transformative journey, seeking to understand the nature of suffering and the path to liberation. After years of rigorous contemplation and meditation, he attained enlightenment under the Bodhi tree.

The Four Noble Truths: The Buddha's teachings on suffering and the path to freedom form the core of Buddhist philosophy. Central to these teachings is the concept of mindfulness. The first of the Four Noble Truths states that suffering exists, but it can be transcended. Mindfulness is the tool by which individuals can become aware of their suffering, its causes, and the path to its cessation.

The Evolution of Mindfulness: From Ancient Traditions to Modern Practice

From its origins in ancient India, mindfulness traveled across cultures and centuries, evolving along the way. It found its home not only in Buddhism but also in various contemplative traditions. Let's explore how mindfulness evolved through the ages.

Early Buddhist Practices: In the early Buddhist scriptures mindfulness was referred to as "sati" in Pali or "smṛti" in Sanskrit It was described as the practice of awareness and recollection— remembering to stay present and attentive to one's experiences The Satipatthana Sutta, a foundational text, outlines the Four Foundations of Mindfulness, which include mindfulness of the body, feelings, mind, and mental qualities.

Zen Buddhism: As Buddhism spread to East Asia, particularly in China and Japan, it took on new forms. Zen Buddhism, known for its direct and experiential approach, emphasized mindfulness in the context of meditation (zazen). Zen masters encouraged practitioners to cultivate "shikantaza," or "just sitting," which involved sitting in complete awareness, without striving for any particular outcome.

Taoist Influence: In China, the influence of Taoism, a native spiritual tradition, merged with Buddhist teachings. This fusion gave rise to Chan Buddhism, which later evolved into Zen Buddhism in Japan. Taoist principles of naturalness, simplicity, and harmony influenced the development of mindfulness practices within these traditions.

Mindfulness in the Modern World

In recent decades, mindfulness has undergone a remarkable transformation, transcending its spiritual origins to become a secular and evidence-based practice. The modern mindfulness movement has made this ancient practice accessible to people of all backgrounds, cultures, and belief systems.

Jon Kabat-Zinn and Mindfulness-Based Stress Reduction (MBSR): One of the key figures in the modern mindfulness movement is Jon Kabat-Zinn, a professor of medicine. In the late 1970s, Kabat-Zinn developed the Mindfulness-Based Stress Reduction (MBSR) program at the University of Massachusetts Medical School. MBSR was designed to help individuals cope with chronic pain and stress using mindfulness techniques. It marked a significant shift in how mindfulness was perceived, as it was stripped of its religious connotations and presented as a practical tool for well-being.

Mindfulness-Based Cognitive Therapy (MBCT): Building on the success of MBSR, Mindfulness-Based Cognitive Therapy (MBCT) was developed as a treatment for depression. MBCT integrates mindfulness practices with principles of cognitive therapy to prevent relapse in individuals with recurrent depression. It has since gained recognition in the field of mental health.

Scientific Research: In recent years, mindfulness has garnered considerable attention from researchers and scientists. Studies have explored its impact on mental health, physical well-being, and cognitive function. This scientific scrutiny has led to the recognition of mindfulness as a valuable tool for stress reduction, emotional regulation, and overall psychological resilience.

C. Mindfulness in Today's Fast-Paced World

In the whirlwind of the modern world, where time races by, demands pile up, and the digital age constantly beckons for our attention, the practice of mindfulness stands as an oasis of calm and clarity. It offers a profound counterbalance to the relentless pace and the ceaseless distractions that define our lives as busy professionals. In this section, we'll explore the relevance and significance of mindfulness in today's fast-paced world.

The Acceleration of Modern Life

Never before in human history has life moved at such a rapid pace. The 21st century has ushered in a wave of technological advancements, transforming the way we work, communicate, and live. While these advancements have brought unprecedented convenience and connectivity, they've also accelerated the pace of life.

Digital Distractions: The digital age has brought with it a constant stream of notifications, emails, and messages. Our smartphones, once hailed as tools of convenience, have become sources of distraction that often hijack our attention. We're constantly pulled in multiple directions, toggling between work, social media, news updates, and personal messages.

Information Overload: The internet has granted us access to a vast sea of information, but it's also overwhelmed us with data. The sheer volume of information can lead to cognitive overload, leaving us feeling overwhelmed and mentally fatigued.

The 24/7 Work Culture: Many professionals find themselves caught in a 24/7 work culture, where boundaries between work and personal life blur. Emails and work-related tasks can follow us home, encroaching on our precious moments of rest and relaxation.

The Cult of Busyness: Busy has become a badge of honor in today's society. We often equate busyness with productivity and success, but it can come at the cost of our well-being. The constant rush leaves little time for reflection, self-care, or simply enjoying the present moment.

The Toll of Modern Life: Stress and Overwhelm

The relentless pace of modern life has given rise to two formidable challenges that impact both our mental and physical well-being: stress and overwhelm.

The Stress Epidemic: Stress has become a ubiquitous companion for many professionals. The pressures of meeting deadlines, achieving targets, and navigating workplace dynamics contribute to chronic stress. The toll of stress on health and happiness is well-documented, leading to a range of physical and mental health issues.

The Burden of Overwhelm: Overwhelm is another common experience. The constant barrage of information and decisions can lead to cognitive overload. We're often faced with a never-ending to-do list and a sense of being stretched too thin. This state of overwhelm affects our ability to think clearly and make effective decisions.

The Role of Mindfulness in the Modern World

In the midst of this frenetic pace and the challenges it brings, mindfulness emerges as a profound antidote. It's not a retreat from the modern world, but a way to navigate it more skillfully. Let's explore how mindfulness is not only relevant but essential in today's fast-paced world.

Cultivating Presence in a World of Distraction

Mindfulness is about cultivating presence—the ability to be fully aware of the present moment. In a world where distraction is the norm, mindfulness teaches us to anchor our attention to the here and now. It's a practice of coming back to ourselves, like finding a quiet sanctuary amidst the noise.

Digital Detox: Mindfulness encourages us to unplug from the constant stream of digital distractions. By being fully present in our activities, whether it's a work task, a conversation with a colleague, or a moment of solitude, we reclaim our attention and regain a sense of control over our lives.

Enhanced Focus: Mindfulness sharpens our focus—a valuable skill in an age of information overload. It teaches us to concentrate on one task at a time, rather than succumbing to the allure of multitasking. This heightened focus allows us to work more efficiently and make better decisions.

Stress Reduction and Emotional Resilience

Mindfulness offers a powerful means to combat stress and build emotional resilience. It equips us with the tools to respond to stressors with composure and clarity.

Stress Reduction: Mindfulness practices, such as deep breathing and meditation, activate the body's relaxation response. They reduce the production of stress hormones, helping us find relief from the pressures of daily life.

Emotional Regulation: Mindfulness enhances emotional intelligence. It teaches us to observe our emotions without judgment and respond to them skillfully. Rather than reacting impulsively, we gain the capacity to pause and choose our responses thoughtfully.

Mindfulness and Well-Being

In a world where busyness is celebrated, mindfulness invites us to prioritize well-being. It encourages self-care, self-compassion, and a deeper connection with ourselves.

Self-Care: Mindfulness reminds us of the importance of self-care. It encourages us to take breaks, engage in relaxation techniques, and nourish our bodies with mindful eating. These practices replenish our energy and prevent burnout.

Self-Compassion: Mindfulness fosters self-compassion. It teaches us to treat ourselves with kindness and understanding, especially in moments of difficulty or failure. This self-compassion is a powerful buffer against the harsh self-criticism that often accompanies the pursuit of perfection.

The Mindful Professional: Navigating Work and Life

Mindfulness is not just a personal practice; it's a professional asset. In the workplace, it equips us with essential skills for success.

Conflict Resolution: Mindfulness enhances our capacity for empathetic listening and open communication. It helps us navigate conflicts and build harmonious relationships with colleagues and clients.

Decision-Making: Mindfulness sharpens our decision-making skills. By approaching decisions with a calm and clear mind, we're more likely to make choices aligned with our values and goals.

Resilience: Mindfulness cultivates resilience—the ability to bounce back from setbacks. It teaches us to view challenges as opportunities for growth and learning, rather than insurmountable obstacles.

The Mindfulness Revolution

The recognition of mindfulness's significance in the professional world has led to a mindfulness revolution. It's not confined to meditation retreats or yoga studios; it's happening in boardrooms, classrooms, and office cubicles.

Corporate Mindfulness Programs: Major corporations, including Google, General Mills, and Salesforce, have introduced mindfulness programs for employees. These programs aim to enhance well-being, reduce stress, and boost productivity.

Education and Healthcare: Mindfulness has found its way into education and healthcare. Schools and universities offer mindfulness courses to help students manage stress and improve focus. Healthcare providers incorporate mindfulness-based interventions into mental health treatment.

Embracing Mindfulness in Today's Fast-Paced World

As you navigate the pages of this ebook, you'll discover practical strategies and techniques to integrate mindfulness seamlessly into your busy professional life. You'll learn how to find moments of calm amidst the chaos, how to cultivate greater focus in the digital age, and how to build resilience in the face of stress and overwhelm.

Mindfulness is not an escape from the modern world, but a companion that helps you thrive within it. It's a timeless practice that has found renewed relevance in our fast-paced era—a practice that empowers you to engage with life more fully, to find serenity in the midst of chaos, and to discover the profound wisdom that resides within each mindful moment.

Are you ready to embrace mindfulness as your ally in the modern world? The journey awaits, and the benefits are profound. Let's explore the path of "On-the-Go Mindfulness" together.

CHAPTER-2

THE MINDFUL MINDSET FOR PROFESSIONALS

In this chapter, we delve into the essential components of the mindful mindset for professionals. We'll explore the unique challenges faced by busy professionals in today's fast-paced world, the detrimental impact of stress on both performance and well-being, and the distinct advantage that a mindful approach offers in navigating the demands of a professional life.

A. The Unique Challenges of Busy Professionals

Busy professionals inhabit a unique and often demanding ecosystem. Whether you're in a corporate office, a healthcare setting, an educational institution, or any other professional field, you're likely familiar with the particular challenges that come with your role. Let's take a closer look at these challenges and why they call for a mindful approach.

Time Constraints: Professionals often grapple with tight schedules and looming deadlines. The pressure to accomplish tasks efficiently can lead to a constant sense of urgency and an overreliance on multitasking.

Digital Overload: The digital age has revolutionized the way professionals work, but it has also inundated them with a relentless stream of emails, messages, and notifications. This continuous connectivity can blur the boundaries between work and personal life.

High Expectations: Professional roles often come with high expectations—expectations of productivity, performance, and meeting targets. The pursuit of excellence can sometimes lead to perfectionism and self-imposed stress.

Complex Decision-Making: Many professionals are tasked with making complex decisions that can have far-reaching consequences. The weight of these decisions can contribute to anxiety and mental fatigue.

B. The Impact of Stress on Performance and Well-being

Stress is an unwelcome companion that often accompanies the demands of a professional life. While a certain level of stress can be motivating, chronic and excessive stress takes a toll on both performance and well-being.

Performance Impairment: Prolonged stress can impair cognitive functions such as decision-making, problem-solving, and creative thinking. It can hinder the ability to focus and lead to reduced productivity.

Emotional Toll: Stress can also have a significant emotional impact. It can lead to mood swings, irritability, and a sense of overwhelm. Chronic stress is associated with increased levels of anxiety and depression.

Physical Health Consequences: The effects of stress extend beyond the mind, affecting the body as well. Stress can contribute to a range of physical health issues, including hypertension, cardiovascular problems, digestive disorders, and compromised immune function.

Burnout: In extreme cases, the persistent pressure and stressors of professional life can result in burnout—a state of emotional, mental, and physical exhaustion. Burnout can lead to disengagement from work, a sense of cynicism, and a decline in job satisfaction.

The Mindful Professional Advantage

Amidst these challenges and the perils of stress, the mindful professional enjoys a distinct advantage. Mindfulness equips professionals with a set of invaluable tools and a resilient mindset that can make all the difference in navigating the complexities of their roles.

Enhanced Focus and Clarity: Mindfulness cultivates heightened awareness and concentration. This enhanced focus allows professionals to approach their tasks with clarity, reducing the likelihood of errors and promoting effective decision-making.

Emotional Resilience: Mindfulness fosters emotional resilience, enabling professionals to respond to stressors with equanimity. Rather than reacting impulsively to difficult situations, they learn to pause and choose their responses thoughtfully.

Stress Reduction: Mindfulness practices, such as meditation and deep breathing, activate the body's relaxation response. They reduce the production of stress hormones, providing professionals with a valuable tool for stress reduction and emotional regulation.

Improved Interpersonal Relationships: Mindfulness enhances interpersonal skills by promoting empathetic listening, open communication, and conflict resolution. Professionals who practice mindfulness often find that their relationships with colleagues, clients, and superiors improve.

Enhanced Well-being: Ultimately, mindfulness contributes to enhanced overall well-being. It encourages self-care, self-compassion, and a deeper connection with oneself. Mindful professionals are better equipped to maintain a sense of balance and fulfillment in their lives.

In the chapters that follow, we'll delve deeper into the practical strategies and techniques that allow professionals to infuse mindfulness into their daily lives. We'll explore how to apply mindfulness in the workplace, during the daily commute, and even in those brief moments of respite during the day. As we do so, you'll gain a comprehensive understanding of how the mindful mindset and practices can truly transform your professional life. It's a journey towards greater clarity, presence, and well-being in the midst of your demanding professional world.

CHAPTER-3

EMBRACING MIDFULNESS: GETTING STARTED

In this chapter, we embark on the practical journey of embracing mindfulness. We'll explore the steps to prepare yourself for mindfulness, the essential mindfulness mindset, and the creation of your mindful space.

A. Preparing Yourself for Mindfulness

Before diving into mindfulness practices, it's essential to prepare yourself mentally and emotionally for this transformative journey. Here are some key aspects to consider:

Openness to Experience: Mindfulness begins with an open attitude. Be willing to explore your inner world with curiosity and without judgment. Approach your experiences with a sense of wonder, as if you're encountering them for the first time.

Commitment and Consistency: Mindfulness is most effective when practiced consistently. Set aside dedicated time for your mindfulness practice, even if it's just a few minutes each day. Consistency builds the habit of mindfulness.

Patience with Yourself: Understand that mindfulness is a skill that develops over time. You might encounter moments of frustration or restlessness during your practice. Approach these moments with patience and self-compassion.

Expectations and Goals: Let go of preconceived expectations and goals for your mindfulness practice. Instead of striving for a particular outcome, focus on the process of being present. Mindfulness is about the journey, not the destination.

B. The Mindfulness Mindset

The mindfulness mindset is a set of qualities and attitudes that form the foundation of your practice. Cultivating these attributes can greatly enhance your experience of mindfulness:

Non-Judgment: Approach your thoughts, emotions, and sensations without judgment. Instead of labeling them as good or bad, simply observe them as they arise. This non-judgmental stance creates a space for self-acceptance.

Beginner's Mind: Cultivate a "beginner's mind," which means approaching each moment with fresh eyes and an open heart. Let go of assumptions and preconceptions, and see things as if for the first time.

Patience: Mindfulness requires patience. Be patient with yourself as you learn and grow in your practice. Understand that moments of distraction or restlessness are a natural part of the process.

Acceptance and Compassion: Practice self-acceptance and self-compassion. Treat yourself with the same kindness and understanding that you would offer to a dear friend. Embrace your imperfections and vulnerabilities.

Letting Go: Mindfulness involves letting go of attachments and clinging. This includes letting go of the past and the future, and fully inhabiting the present moment. It also means letting go of the need to control or manipulate your experiences.

C. Creating Your Mindful Space

Creating a mindful space is an essential aspect of integrating mindfulness into your daily life. Here's how to establish a conducive environment for your practice:

Select a Quiet Space: Choose a quiet and comfortable space where you won't be easily disturbed. It could be a corner of your home, a quiet park bench, or even a spot in your office where you can find moments of solitude.

Reduce Distractions: Minimize external distractions in your chosen space. Turn off notifications on your devices, close the door if necessary, and create an environment that supports your focus.

Comfortable Seating: Select a chair, cushion, or mat that allows you to sit comfortably for the duration of your practice. The goal is to maintain a posture that is both alert and relaxed.

Nurturing Elements: Consider adding elements that nurture your senses, such as soft lighting, a soothing color palette, or a plant. These elements can create a sense of tranquility in your space.

Personal Touches: Infuse your mindful space with personal touches that resonate with you. It could be a meaningful quote, a piece of art, or a symbol that represents mindfulness to you.

As you prepare yourself for mindfulness, embrace the mindfulness mindset, and create your mindful space, you'll be setting a strong foundation for your practice. In the chapters ahead, we'll delve into specific mindfulness techniques and exercises that you can incorporate into your daily routine, bringing mindfulness to life in your busy professional world.

CHAPTER-4

QUICK MINDFULNESS PRACTICES FOR BUSY SCHEDULES

In this chapter, we explore "Mindful Moments," a collection of quick mindfulness practices designed to fit seamlessly into your busy schedule. These practices offer a gateway to presence, calm, and clarity in the midst of a hectic day. We'll begin with an introduction to "Mindful Moments" and then delve into the foundational practice of mindful breathing, followed by mindful mini-meditations and strategies for integrating these practices into your daily routine.

A. Introduction to "Mindful Moments"

In the fast-paced world of busy professionals, finding time for extended mindfulness sessions can be challenging. However, the beauty of mindfulness lies in its adaptability. "Mindful Moments" are designed to be brief yet impactful practices that can be woven into the fabric of your day.

Think of "Mindful Moments" as tiny islands of tranquility amidst the ocean of your responsibilities. These moments allow you to pause, breathe, and reconnect with the present, even when you're pressed for time. They are like mini-vacations for your mind, offering respite from the busyness of your schedule.

"Mindful Moments" are not about adding more to your to-do list. Instead, they're about optimizing the moments that already exist in your day. Whether you're in a meeting, commuting, or waiting for a coffee, you can use these moments to nurture your well-being and strengthen your mindfulness muscle.

The practices we'll explore in this chapter are versatile, adaptable and easy to learn. They are suitable for both beginners and experienced practitioners. So, if you're ready to infuse your day with moments of mindfulness, let's begin with the foundational practice of mindful breathing.

B. Mindful Breathing: A Foundation for Presence

Mindful breathing is a cornerstone of mindfulness practice. It's a simple yet powerful technique that anchors your attention to the present moment by focusing on your breath. Here's how to cultivate the art of mindful breathing:

1. **Find a Quiet Moment**: While mindful breathing can be practiced anywhere, it's helpful to begin in a quiet space where you can concentrate. You can later incorporate it into busier settings.

2. **Get Comfortable**: Sit in a comfortable yet alert posture. You can be seated on a chair or cushion, or even standing or walking if that's more convenient.

3. **Begin to Breathe**: Close your eyes if you feel comfortable doing so. Start by taking a few deep, intentional breaths. Feel the rise and fall of your chest or the expansion and contraction of your abdomen with each breath.

4. **Focus on the Breath**: Now, shift your attention to the natural rhythm of your breath. Observe the sensation of the breath as it enters and leaves your nostrils or the rise and fall of your abdomen.

5. **Stay Present**: Your mind may wander, and that's perfectly normal. When it does, gently and non-judgmentally bring your attention back to your breath. Think of your breath as an anchor to the present moment.

6. **Set a Timer**: If you're just starting, you can set a timer for a few minutes to guide your practice. As you become more comfortable, you can extend the duration.

Mindful breathing is like a reset button for your mind. It calms the mental chatter, reduces stress, and enhances your ability to respond to situations with greater clarity and composure. Even in the midst of a demanding day, you can take a "Mindful Moment" to practice this foundational technique.

C. Mindful Mini-Meditations: Finding Stillness in Seconds

Mini-meditations are brief mindfulness practices that offer a moment of stillness and reflection, even in the busiest of schedules. These practices can be completed in as little as a minute or two, making them highly accessible.

Here are two examples of mindful mini-meditations:

1. The Breath Awareness Mini-Meditation:

- *Find a quiet space, if possible, or simply close your eyes for a moment.*
- *Take a few deep breaths to settle into the present moment.*
- *Observe your breath as it moves in and out of your body.*
- *With each inhale, silently say to yourself, "I am here."*
- *With each exhale, silently say, "This is now."*

- *Repeat this for a minute or longer if you have the time.*

*2. **The Body Scan Mini-Meditation:***

- *Sit comfortably and close your eyes, if you can.*
- *Begin by bringing your attention to your toes.*
- *Slowly scan up through your feet, ankles, calves, and so on, until you reach the top of your head.*
- *As you scan, notice any areas of tension or discomfort without judgment.*
- *Take a deep breath, and as you exhale, imagine releasing any tension or stress you've identified.*
- *Open your eyes and continue with your day, feeling more relaxed and present.*

These mini-meditations serve as mindful pauses during your day, allowing you to step out of autopilot mode and into a state of awareness. They can be particularly helpful during moments of stress or overwhelm, providing a brief respite to recalibrate and center yourself.

D. Integrating Mindful Moments into Your Day

The beauty of "Mindful Moments" is their adaptability to various situations throughout your day. Here are some strategies for seamlessly integrating these practices into your daily routine:

1. **Morning Mindfulness**: Start your day with a "Mindful Moment." As you wake up, take a few mindful breaths or spend a minute setting a positive intention for the day ahead.

2. **Commuting Calm**: If you commute, use that time for mindfulness. Whether you're driving, cycling, or taking public transport, you can practice mindful breathing or awareness of your surroundings.

3. **Meeting Mindfulness**: In the workplace, use meetings as opportunities for mindfulness. Take a minute before a meeting to center yourself with a few breaths, and practice active listening during the meeting itself.

4. **Lunchtime Reflection**: During lunch breaks, savor your meal mindfully. Pay attention to the flavors, textures, and smells. It's a brief yet nourishing "Mindful Moment."

5. **Nature Connection**: If possible, spend a few moments in nature each day. Whether it's a stroll in the park or a glance at the sky, connect with the natural world around you.

6. **Bedtime Peace**: As you wind down in the evening, take a "Mindful Moment" to reflect on your day. Express gratitude for positive experiences and acknowledge any challenges with self-compassion.

The key to integrating mindfulness into your day is to make it a habit. Start small, and gradually build on these practices as they become more ingrained in your routine. Over time, you'll find that "Mindful Moments" become second nature, providing pockets of calm and clarity in even the busiest of schedules.

CHAPTER-5

MINDFULNESS FOR STRESS REDUCTIONS

In this chapter, we explore the profound impact of mindfulness on stress reduction, a critical aspect of managing the demands of a busy professional life. We'll begin by delving into the insidious nature of stress as a silent productivity killer. Then, we'll explore the science behind how mindfulness can effectively reduce stress. Finally, we'll delve into various mindfulness-based stress reduction techniques that you can incorporate into your daily routine.

A. Stress: The Silent Productivity Killer

Stress is a pervasive and often silent productivity killer that affects countless professionals in today's fast-paced world. It creeps into our lives, disrupts our well-being, and sabotages our ability to perform at our best. Understanding the impact of stress is the first step towards effective stress management.

The Stealthy Nature of Stress: Stress is like a stealthy intruder that gradually infiltrates our lives. It can begin with seemingly minor pressures, such as meeting deadlines or handling a heavy workload. Over time, if left unchecked, it can escalate into chronic stress.

Physical and Emotional Toll: Stress takes a toll on both our physical and emotional well-being. Physically, it can lead to muscle tension, headaches, and digestive problems. Emotionally, it can result in anxiety, irritability, and even depression.

Impaired Cognitive Function: Stress impairs cognitive functions critical for professional success, such as decision-making, problem-solving, and creative thinking. It can lead to mental fatigue and a decline in performance.

Burnout and Decreased Job Satisfaction: Prolonged stress can culminate in burnout—a state of emotional, mental, and physical exhaustion. Burnout is characterized by disengagement from work, a sense of cynicism, and decreased job satisfaction.

Interpersonal Challenges: **Stress** can strain interpersonal relationships. It may lead to conflicts with colleagues and clients, further exacerbating workplace challenges.

B. The Science of Mindfulness and Stress Reduction

The science behind mindfulness and stress reduction is compelling and offers insights into why this practice is so effective in managing stress.

Stress and the Brain: Stress activates the brain's "fight or flight" response, releasing stress hormones like cortisol and adrenaline. Chronic stress can lead to an overactive stress response, which is detrimental to health.

Mindfulness and the Brain: Mindfulness practices, such as mindful breathing and meditation, have been shown to have a significant impact on the brain. Studies using neuroimaging have revealed that regular mindfulness practice can lead to structural changes in areas of the brain associated with stress regulation, emotional control, and attention.

Reducing the Stress Response: Mindfulness promotes the relaxation response, which counteracts the stress response. It reduces the production of stress hormones and encourages a state of calm and well-being.

Emotional Regulation: Mindfulness enhances emotional regulation. It helps individuals become more aware of their emotional responses and allows them to respond to stressors with greater composure and clarity.

Improved Cognitive Function: Mindfulness improves cognitive functions, including attention, concentration, and decision-making. This is especially important in the face of stress, as it enhances one's ability to think clearly and make effective choices.

C. Mindfulness-Based Stress Reduction Techniques

Mindfulness-based stress reduction techniques are practical tools and practices that you can incorporate into your daily life to effectively manage and reduce stress.

Mindful Breathing: Mindful breathing involves paying attention to your breath as it naturally occurs. By focusing on your breath, you can anchor your attention to the present moment, calm your mind, and reduce stress.

Body Scan Meditation: In a body scan meditation, you systematically focus your attention on different parts of your body, starting from your toes and moving up to your head. This practice promotes relaxation and helps release physical tension.

Mindful Walking: Mindful walking involves walking slowly and deliberately while paying attention to each step and your surroundings. It's an excellent practice for reducing stress and enhancing mindfulness during everyday activities.

Mindful Eating: Mindful eating encourages you to savor each bite of your meal, paying attention to the flavors, textures, and sensations. It promotes a healthier relationship with food and reduces stress related to eating.

Mindful Journaling: Journaling can be a powerful tool for stress reduction. By writing down your thoughts and feelings with self-compassion and without judgment, you can gain clarity and reduce emotional stress.

Progressive Muscle Relaxation: This technique involves systematically tensing and then relaxing different muscle groups in your body. It can help alleviate physical tension and promote relaxation.

Guided Mindfulness Meditations: Guided mindfulness meditations are audio recordings led by an instructor. They can provide structured guidance and support for your mindfulness practice, making it easier to incorporate into your routine.

These mindfulness-based stress reduction techniques offer practical ways to manage and reduce stress in your busy professional life. By integrating these practices into your daily routine, you can experience the profound benefits of mindfulness in cultivating resilience, promoting well-being, and enhancing your overall quality of life.

CHAPTER-6

MINDFUL COMMUNICATIONS BUILDING BETTER RELATIONSHIPS

In this chapter, we explore the transformative potential of mindful communication in both personal and professional relationships. We'll begin by understanding the profound power of mindful communication. Then, we'll delve into the art of mindful listening, which is a gift not only to others but also to yourself. Finally, we'll explore how to apply mindful communication principles both at work and in your personal life.

A. The Power of Mindful Communication

Mindful communication is a powerful and transformative practice that goes beyond mere words. It involves being fully present and engaged in your interactions, fostering deeper connections, and creating a more harmonious environment. Here's why mindful communication holds such incredible potential:

Presence and Authenticity: Mindful communication starts with being present in the moment. When you are fully engaged in a conversation, you convey authenticity and sincerity. This presence allows you to truly connect with others.

Enhanced Understanding: Mindful communication involves active listening and open-heartedness. It fosters a deeper understanding of the thoughts, feelings, and perspectives of those you interact with. By truly hearing others, you can bridge gaps in communication and build trust.

***Reduced Conflicts*:** Mindful communication encourages non-reactive responses. Instead of reacting impulsively, you learn to respond thoughtfully, reducing the likelihood of conflicts and misunderstandings.

***Improved Emotional Regulation*:** Mindful communication supports emotional regulation. It helps you manage your own emotions and respond to the emotions of others with empathy and compassion.

***Enhanced Relationships*:** By practicing mindful communication, you can cultivate healthier and more fulfilling relationships, both in your personal life and in the workplace. It contributes to a positive and supportive communication culture.

B. Mindful Listening: A Gift to Others and Yourself

Mindful listening is a cornerstone of effective communication. It involves not only hearing the words spoken but also fully attending to the speaker with an open heart and mind. Here's how mindful listening benefits both you and those you engage with:

***Deep Connection*:** Mindful listening creates a deep connection between you and the speaker. By giving them your full attention, you show that you value and respect their perspective.

***Validation and Empathy*:** When you truly listen, you validate the speaker's feelings and experiences. This validation can foster a sense of trust and empathy in your relationship.

***Reduced Misunderstandings*:** Misunderstandings often arise from incomplete or hasty listening. Mindful listening reduces the chances of misinterpreting what is being communicated.

Conflict Resolution: In conflicts or disagreements, mindful listening is essential. It allows each party to express themselves fully and feel heard, which is a critical step toward finding common ground and resolving issues.

Stress Reduction: Mindful listening can also reduce stress, both for the speaker and the listener. It promotes a sense of being understood and supported, which can alleviate tension.

C. Mindful Communication at Work and Home

Mindful communication is valuable in both professional and personal settings. Here's how you can apply mindful communication principles to enhance relationships at work and at home:

At Work:

1. **Meetings**: Practice mindful communication in meetings by actively listening to colleagues and contributing thoughtfully. Encourage open dialogue and create a culture of respect and collaboration.

2. **Emails and Messages**: Mindful communication extends to written communication as well. Before sending emails or messages, take a moment to consider your tone and the impact of your words.

3. **Conflict Resolution**: When conflicts arise, engage in mindful communication to understand the perspectives of all parties involved. Use empathetic listening and non-reactive responses to navigate disagreements.

At Home:

1. **Family Communication**: Apply mindful communication with your family members. This includes listening to your loved ones without judgment, expressing yourself honestly, and fostering an environment of trust and support.

2. **Parenting**: Mindful communication can be particularly valuable in parenting. Listening attentively to your children's concerns and emotions can strengthen your bond and create a nurturing home environment.

3. **Personal Relationships**: In your personal relationships, prioritize open and honest communication. Use mindful listening to understand your partner's needs and feelings, and express your own thoughts and emotions with care.

4. **Conflict Resolution**: Just as in the workplace, mindful communication is essential for resolving conflicts within your family or personal relationships. Approach disagreements with patience, empathy, and a willingness to find common ground.

By integrating mindful communication into your daily interactions, you can experience profound improvements in your relationships, whether at work or at home. Mindful listening, empathy, and authenticity are powerful tools that can lead to deeper connections, reduced conflicts, and a more harmonious and fulfilling life.

CHAPTER-7

BUILDING RESILINECE THROUGH MINDFULNESS

In this chapter, we explore how mindfulness can play a pivotal role in building resilience, a valuable skill for navigating life's challenges and setbacks. We'll begin by understanding the fundamental role of mindfulness in resilience. Then, we'll delve into practical strategies for bouncing back from setbacks. Finally, we'll explore how mindfulness can help you cultivate a positive mindset that fosters resilience.

A. The Role of Mindfulness in Building Resilience

Mindfulness serves as a foundational pillar in the development of resilience—a crucial capacity for effectively coping with adversity and maintaining well-being. Here's why mindfulness is integral to building resilience:

Emotional Regulation: Mindfulness equips you with the ability to observe and regulate your emotions. When faced with challenging situations, you can remain composed and make thoughtful decisions instead of reacting impulsively.

Stress Reduction: Mindfulness practices reduce stress and the harmful effects it can have on your physical and mental health. By mitigating stress, mindfulness enhances your resilience in the face of adversity.

Adaptive Responses: Mindfulness encourages adaptive responses to difficulties. Instead of dwelling on negative thoughts or getting overwhelmed, you can approach problems with a clear and balanced perspective.

Enhanced Problem-Solving: Mindfulness enhances cognitive functions, including problem-solving and decision-making. These skills are essential for overcoming obstacles and finding effective solutions.

Self-Compassion: Mindfulness fosters self-compassion, allowing you to treat yourself with kindness and understanding during challenging times. This self-compassion is a powerful tool for building resilience.

B. Strategies for Bouncing Back from Setbacks

Resilience involves the ability to bounce back from setbacks and adapt positively to adversity. Mindfulness can help you develop and strengthen this resilience. Here are practical strategies for bouncing back from setbacks:

Acceptance of Reality: Mindfulness encourages acceptance of the present moment, including acknowledging setbacks and difficulties without judgment. This acceptance is the first step toward resilience.

Self-Reflection: Engage in self-reflection to gain insights from setbacks. Mindfulness provides a space for introspection, helping you understand your reactions and learn from your experiences.

Optimism and Realism: Cultivate an optimistic yet realistic mindset. While it's essential to maintain a positive outlook, it's equally important to acknowledge and address challenges realistically.

Positive Coping Mechanisms: Mindfulness promotes the use of positive coping mechanisms, such as seeking social support, problem-solving, and self-care, when faced with setbacks.

Emotional Resilience: Develop emotional resilience by allowing yourself to feel and process emotions associated with setbacks. Mindfulness can help you navigate these emotions in a healthy way.

Flexibility and Adaptability: Resilience involves flexibility and adaptability. Mindfulness cultivates these qualities by encouraging you to remain open to change and new possibilities.

C. Cultivating a Positive Mindset

Cultivating a positive mindset through mindfulness is a proactive way to bolster resilience. Here's how you can use mindfulness to foster positivity:

Gratitude Practice: Engage in regular gratitude practices to shift your focus toward positive aspects of your life. Mindfulness allows you to fully savor and appreciate the present moment.

Positive Affirmations: Incorporate positive affirmations into your daily routine. Mindfulness helps you internalize these affirmations and challenge negative self-talk.

Mindful Self-Compassion: Treat yourself with kindness and self-compassion. Mindfulness encourages self-care and self-nurturing which are essential for maintaining a positive mindset.

Focus on Strengths: Use mindfulness to identify and leverage your strengths. Recognizing your capabilities can boost your self-esteem and confidence.

Positive Visualization: Engage in positive visualization exercises, where you imagine successful outcomes and achievements. Mindfulness can enhance the effectiveness of these visualizations.

Resilience-Building Mindfulness Practices: Incorporate specific mindfulness practices that focus on building resilience. These practices may include mindful breathing, body scans, or meditation.

By integrating these strategies into your life and practicing mindfulness consistently, you can build resilience that equips you to face adversity with grace and adaptability. Resilience not only helps you overcome setbacks but also fosters personal growth and enhances your overall well-being.

CHAPTER-8

MINDFUL TECH USE IN DIGITAL WORLD

In this chapter, we explore the challenges posed by the digital age and how mindfulness can be harnessed to navigate the complexities of technology in a more balanced and productive manner. We'll begin by delving into the dilemmas presented by the digital age. Then, we'll explore practical mindful tech practices that enhance productivity. Finally, we'll discuss strategies for reclaiming your time and attention from the demands of the digital world.

A. The Digital Age Dilemma

The digital age has ushered in unprecedented advancements and conveniences, but it has also given rise to challenges that affect our well-being and productivity. Here are some of the dilemmas posed by the digital age:

Information Overload: The constant stream of information and notifications can lead to information overload, making it challenging to focus on important tasks.

Digital Distractions: The allure of social media, entertainment, and endless apps can be highly distracting, pulling our attention away from meaningful work and real-life experiences.

Fragmented Attention: Multitasking, a common practice in the digital age, can fragment our attention, reduce productivity, and hinder deep work.

Screen Fatigue: Excessive screen time can lead to physical discomfort, eye strain, and mental fatigue.

Diminished Face-to-Face Connections: Overreliance on digital communication can erode face-to-face social interactions and interpersonal skills.

B. Mindful Tech Practices for Greater Productivity

Mindfulness can be a powerful tool for harnessing technology to enhance productivity. Here are practical mindful tech practices that can help you use digital tools more intentionally:

Digital Detox: Periodically disconnect from digital devices to reset and recharge. Use this time to engage in offline activities, connect with nature, or practice mindfulness.

Set Tech Boundaries: Establish clear boundaries for tech use. Designate specific times for checking emails and social media, and stick to these boundaries.

Single-Tasking: Practice single-tasking rather than multitasking. Give your full attention to one task at a time to enhance focus and productivity.

Digital Mindfulness Reminders: Set reminders on your devices to prompt mindful pauses throughout the day. Use these reminders to check in with your breath, posture, and overall well-being.

Tech-Free Zones: Designate certain areas or times as tech-free zones. For example, create a tech-free bedroom to improve sleep quality.

App and Notification Management: Review and minimize the number of apps and notifications on your devices. Disable non-essential notifications to reduce distractions.

Mindful Tech Use: Before engaging with technology, pause for a moment of mindfulness. Ask yourself if the digital activity aligns with your goals and values.

C. Reclaiming Your Time and Attention

Reclaiming your time and attention in the digital age is essential for personal well-being and productivity. Here are strategies to help you regain control:

Prioritize Digital Activities: Identify the most meaningful and productive digital activities in your life. Allocate your time and attention accordingly.

Create a Tech-Free Routine: Establish a tech-free routine in the morning or evening to allow for more mindful and intentional starts and endings to your day.

Implement Digital Sprints: Use the Pomodoro Technique or similar time management methods to work in focused, timed intervals with short breaks. This approach can boost productivity and attention.

Practice Digital Mindfulness: Cultivate mindfulness when using technology. Pay attention to your intentions, emotions, and physical sensations while engaging with digital devices.

Digital Curfew: Set a digital curfew, restricting tech use during a specific time in the evening to promote better sleep and relaxation

Regular Tech Assessments: Periodically assess your digital habits and make adjustments to align them with your goals and values.

Tech-Free Leisure Activities: Incorporate tech-free leisure activities into your routine. Engage in hobbies, exercise, or simply relax without the constant presence of screens.

By implementing these strategies and practicing mindfulness in your interactions with technology, you can reclaim your time and attention, reduce digital distractions, and use digital tools in a more purposeful and balanced way. This approach allows you to harness the benefits of the digital age while maintaining your well-being and productivity.

CHAPTER-9
REAL-LIFE SUCCESS STORIES

In this inspiring chapter, we share real-life success stories of professionals who have experienced transformative changes in their careers and lives through the practice of mindfulness. These stories illustrate the tangible impact of mindfulness on personal and professional growth. We'll begin by delving into stories of transformation, highlighting the real professionals and their remarkable journeys. Then, we'll explore how mindfulness has changed their careers and lives for the better.

A. Stories of Transformation: Real Professionals, Real Results

The stories of transformation featured in this section showcase the experiences of real professionals who have harnessed the power of mindfulness to bring about positive change in their lives. These individuals come from diverse backgrounds and face a range of challenges, but they share a common thread—the profound impact of mindfulness on their personal and professional journeys.

From Burnout to Balance: Meet Sarah, a dedicated healthcare professional who was on the brink of burnout. Through mindfulness practices, she learned to prioritize self-care, set boundaries, and find balance in her demanding career.

Overcoming Impostor Syndrome: John, an ambitious young entrepreneur, battled impostor syndrome and self-doubt as he navigated the competitive business world. Mindfulness helped him cultivate self-confidence, resilience, and a growth mindset.

Enhancing Leadership Skills: Lisa, a corporate executive, sought to improve her leadership skills and foster a more inclusive workplace culture. Mindfulness practices equipped her with the emotional intelligence and presence needed to lead with compassion and authenticity.

Managing Chronic Stress: David, a high-achieving lawyer, faced chronic stress and anxiety that threatened his well-being. Mindfulness meditation became his anchor, enabling him to manage stress effectively and maintain mental clarity.

Career Transition and Clarity: Michelle, a mid-career professional, found herself at a crossroads and uncertain about her career direction. Mindfulness facilitated self-discovery, helping her gain clarity and confidence to pursue a new and fulfilling path.

B. How Mindfulness Changed Their Careers and Lives

In this section, we explore how mindfulness has led to transformative changes in the careers and lives of the individuals featured in the success stories. Their journeys exemplify the profound ways in which mindfulness can empower personal and professional growth.

Enhanced Well-Being: Sarah's story illustrates how mindfulness not only prevented burnout but also enhanced her overall well-being. By prioritizing self-care and practicing mindfulness, she regained vitality and passion for her work.

Increased Confidence and Resilience: John's journey highlights how mindfulness boosted his self-confidence and resilience, allowing him to tackle challenges with a newfound sense of capability and adaptability.

Authentic Leadership: Lisa's experience demonstrates how mindfulness helped her become a more authentic and effective leader. By cultivating empathy and presence, she fostered a workplace culture of inclusivity and collaboration.

Stress Management and Clarity: David's story showcases the impact of mindfulness on stress management and mental clarity. Through mindfulness, he found the tools to alleviate chronic stress and make informed decisions in his legal career.

Career Transformation: Michelle's journey exemplifies how mindfulness can facilitate career transformation. By delving into self-reflection and mindfulness practices, she gained the clarity and courage to transition into a more fulfilling profession.

These real-life success stories serve as powerful testimonies to the potential of mindfulness to reshape careers and lives. They illustrate how mindfulness can empower individuals to overcome challenges, enhance well-being, and unlock their full potential in both their professional endeavors and personal journeys.

CHAPTER-10
CREATING YOUR MINDFUL LIFESTYLE

In this final chapter, we bring together the key insights and practices from the previous chapters to help you create your mindful lifestyle. We'll begin by summarizing the journey you've undertaken so far. Then, we'll guide you through the step-by-step process of crafting your own mindful lifestyle plan. Finally, we'll emphasize the importance of mindfulness as a lifelong companion on your personal and professional journey.

A. Summarizing the Journey So Far

Before embarking on the practical journey of creating your mindful lifestyle, it's essential to reflect on the insights and practices you've encountered in this ebook. Here, we summarize the key takeaways from your journey:

Understanding Mindfulness: You've gained a deep understanding of mindfulness—what it is and how it can benefit busy professionals like yourself. Mindfulness is not just a buzzword; it's a powerful practice that can enhance your well-being, resilience, and productivity.

Mindful Mindset: You've explored the mindful mindset, which involves being fully present, non-judgmental, and compassionate. This mindset forms the foundation for incorporating mindfulness into your daily life.

Practical Techniques: Throughout the ebook, you've discovered practical mindfulness techniques, from mindful breathing to body scans, that you can integrate into your routine. These techniques provide you with tools to manage stress, enhance focus, and cultivate self-awareness.

Enhanced Communication: Mindfulness extends beyond personal well-being; it can also improve your communication and relationships. You've learned how mindful listening and communication can transform your interactions at work and in your personal life.

Building Resilience: Mindfulness is a key factor in building resilience. By regulating emotions, managing stress, and fostering a positive mindset, you're better equipped to navigate life's challenges.

Tech and Digital Balance: In the digital age, you've explored strategies to maintain a healthy balance with technology. Mindful tech practices and setting boundaries are essential for a more focused and fulfilling life.

B. Your Mindful Lifestyle Plan: Step-by-Step

Creating a mindful lifestyle plan is an intentional and transformative process. This step-by-step guide will help you craft a personalized plan that aligns with your goals and integrates mindfulness into your daily life. Mindfulness is not just a practice but a way of living that can enhance your well-being, resilience, and overall quality of life.

Step 1: Define Your Goals

The first step in creating your mindful lifestyle plan is to define your goals. What do you hope to achieve through mindfulness?

Take time to reflect on both your personal and professional aspirations. Are you seeking stress reduction, enhanced focus, improved relationships, or personal growth?

Consider writing down your goals in a journal or on a piece of paper. Having a clear understanding of your objectives will provide direction and motivation as you embark on your mindfulness journey.

Step 2: Choose Your Practices

Mindfulness offers a diverse range of practices, from meditation to mindful eating. Once you've identified your goals, choose mindfulness practices that resonate with you and align with your objectives. Here are some common mindfulness practices to consider:

- **Mindful Breathing**: Focus on your breath to anchor yourself in the present moment and calm your mind.
- **Meditation**: Dedicate time each day to formal meditation, whether it's guided or self-guided.
- **Body Scan**: Pay attention to physical sensations in your body to increase awareness and release tension.
- **Mindful Walking**: Practice walking slowly and attentively, fully experiencing each step.
- **Mindful Eating**: Savor your meals by eating slowly and mindfully, paying attention to taste, texture, and the act of eating itself.
- **Mindful Journaling**: Write down your thoughts and feelings with self-compassion and without judgment.
- **Gratitude Practice**: Cultivate gratitude by reflecting on things you're thankful for in your life.

Step 3: Establish a Routine

Consistency is key to reaping the benefits of mindfulness. Once you've chosen your practices, establish a routine that incorporates mindfulness into your daily or weekly schedule. Consider the following tips:

- Set aside dedicated time: Allocate specific slots in your day for mindfulness practices. This could be in the morning, during breaks, or before bedtime.
- Create reminders: Use alarms, notifications, or mindfulness apps to remind you to engage in your chosen practices.
- Make it a habit: Repetition is essential for building habits. Commit to practicing mindfulness regularly until it becomes a natural part of your routine.

Step 4: Set Intentions

Before each mindfulness practice, set clear intentions. What do you hope to achieve or cultivate through this practice? Setting intentions adds depth and purpose to your mindfulness experience. For example:

- If you're practicing mindful breathing, your intention might be to calm your mind and reduce stress.
- In meditation, your intention could be to increase self-awareness and cultivate inner peace.
- When practicing mindful listening, set an intention to fully hear and understand the person you're engaging with.

Intentions guide your practice and provide a sense of direction. They help you connect with the specific goals you identified in Step 1.

Step 5: Mindful Moments

Incorporate "Mindful Moments" throughout your day. These are brief pauses during which you check in with your breath, posture, and present moment awareness. Mindful moments can be particularly valuable in high-stress situations or when you need to recenter yourself during a busy day.

To integrate mindful moments into your life:

- Choose triggers: Identify cues that remind you to pause and be mindful. For example, you could use the sound of a ringing phone, the act of opening a door, or the sensation of taking a deep breath.
- Keep it brief: Mindful moments don't need to be time-consuming. A few seconds of focused attention can make a significant difference in your overall mindfulness.
- Practice gratitude: Use mindful moments to express gratitude for the present moment and all that it offers.

Step 6: Reflect and Adjust

Regularly reflect on your mindfulness journey. Take time to assess your progress, challenges, and the impact of mindfulness on your life. Journaling can be a powerful tool for self-reflection. Ask yourself questions like:

- What benefits have I experienced from my mindfulness practice?

- Have I noticed changes in my well-being, relationships, or work since I started practicing mindfulness?
- What challenges have I encountered, and how can I address them?
- Are there any adjustments I need to make to my mindfulness routine or goals?

By reflecting on your mindfulness journey, you can adapt and refine your plan to better align with your evolving needs and aspirations. Flexibility and self-compassion are essential components of a sustainable mindfulness practice.

Creating a mindful lifestyle plan is a thoughtful and empowering process that allows you to integrate mindfulness into your daily life. By defining your goals, choosing practices, establishing a routine, setting intentions, incorporating mindful moments, and reflecting on your journey, you can cultivate a mindful way of living that enhances your overall well-being and supports your personal and professional growth. Remember that mindfulness is a lifelong journey, and your plan can evolve as you continue to explore and deepen your practice.

C. Mindfulness as a Lifelong Companion

Lastly, remember that mindfulness is not a destination; it's a lifelong journey and companion. Here's how mindfulness can continue to enrich your life:

Growth and Evolution: As you continue your mindfulness practice, you'll experience personal growth and evolution. Mindfulness deepens your self-awareness and supports ongoing self-improvement.

Resilience and Adaptability: Mindfulness equips you with the resilience and adaptability needed to navigate life's twists and turns. It's a valuable resource for both personal and professional challenges.

Enhanced Well-Being: Mindfulness contributes to your overall well-being. It promotes mental clarity, emotional balance, and physical health, allowing you to lead a more fulfilling life.

Relationships and Connection: Mindfulness enhances your relationships by improving your communication, empathy, and presence. It fosters deeper connections with others.

Professional Success: In your professional life, mindfulness can boost productivity, creativity, and leadership skills. It can also help you manage stress and maintain work-life balance.

Joy and Gratitude: Mindfulness invites you to savor life's moments, find joy in the everyday, and cultivate gratitude. It allows you to appreciate the richness of life.

Embark on your mindful lifestyle journey, remember that mindfulness is a lifelong practice. Embrace it as a trusted companion that supports your growth, resilience, well-being, and personal and professional success. Your mindful lifestyle has the potential to enrich every facet of your life, leading to greater fulfillment and happiness.

CONCLUSION

In this concluding chapter, we embrace the enduring power of mindfulness. As we bid farewell to "On-the-Go Mindfulness," we reflect on the journey you've undertaken and the transformative potential that mindfulness carries into your life.

A. The Power of Mindfulness: A Lasting Legacy

In this concluding chapter, we reflect on the profound power of mindfulness and its potential to leave a lasting legacy in your life. Throughout "On-the-Go Mindfulness," you've embarked on a transformative journey, discovering how mindfulness can enhance your well-being, resilience, and overall quality of life.

Mindfulness is not just a practice; it's a way of living that empowers you to be fully present, cultivate self-awareness, and embrace life's challenges with grace and resilience. By incorporating mindfulness into your daily routine, you've unlocked a powerful tool for personal and professional growth.

As you continue your mindfulness journey, remember that the benefits of mindfulness extend beyond yourself. By enhancing your well-being and relationships, you have the potential to inspire and positively impact those around you. Your mindful legacy can create a ripple effect of positivity and growth in your personal and professional spheres.

B. Embarking on Your Mindfulness Journey

Your mindfulness journey doesn't end with this ebook—it's just the beginning. As you close these pages, take a moment to reflect on the insights, practices, and stories you've encountered. Consider how you can apply mindfulness to your unique circumstances and goals.

Mindfulness is a lifelong practice, and each day presents an opportunity to deepen your awareness and presence. Embrace the challenges and triumphs of your journey, knowing that mindfulness is a trusted companion that can enrich every facet of your life.

C. Thank You for Choosing "On-the-Go Mindfulness"

We extend our heartfelt gratitude for choosing "On-the-Go Mindfulness" as your companion on this transformative journey. We hope this ebook has provided you with valuable insights, practical tools, and inspiration to incorporate mindfulness into your busy professional life.

As you continue to explore the profound benefits of mindfulness, may you find inner peace, enhanced well-being, and a deeper connection to the world around you. Thank you for allowing us to be a part of your mindfulness journey, and may your path be filled with mindfulness, growth, and lasting fulfillment.

ADDITIONAL RESOURCES

As you continue your mindfulness journey, we've compiled a list of valuable resources to support and deepen your practice. These recommended books, websites, and apps provide a wealth of knowledge, guided meditations, and expert insights to enhance your mindfulness experience. Explore these resources to further enrich your understanding and application of mindfulness in your daily life.

Books:

1. "The Miracle of Mindfulness" by Thich Nhat Hanh
2. "Wherever You Go, There You Are" by Jon Kabat-Zinn
3. "The Power of Now" by Eckhart Tolle
4. "Radical Acceptance" by Tara Brach
5. "The Untethered Soul" by Michael A. Singer

Websites:

1. **Mindful.org:** Mindful.org offers articles, guided meditations, and resources to deepen your mindfulness practice.
2. **Greater Good Science Center:** The Greater Good Science Center at UC Berkeley provides research-based articles and practices for well-being, including mindfulness.
3. **Insight Timer:** This website and app offer a vast library of guided meditations and mindfulness courses from various teachers.

4. **Mindfulness-Based Stress Reduction (MBSR):** Explore the official website of MBSR, founded by Jon Kabat-Zinn, for information on mindfulness courses and resources.

Apps:

1. **Headspace:** Headspace offers guided meditations, mindfulness exercises, and sleep aids to improve your overall well-being.

2. **Calm:** Calm provides guided meditations, relaxation techniques, and sleep stories to reduce stress and enhance mindfulness.

3. **10% Happier:** This app features mindfulness courses and teachings from leading meditation teachers and experts.

4. **Insight Timer:** The Insight Timer app offers a vast library of free guided meditations and a supportive community of meditators.

5. **Buddhify:** Buddhify offers mindfulness practices tailored to various aspects of your daily life, making it easy to integrate mindfulness into your busy schedule.

These resources are just a starting point for your ongoing mindfulness journey. Explore, experiment, and discover the resources that resonate most with you. Mindfulness is a personal and evolving practice, and these tools can help you continue to reap its benefits in your life.

ABOUT THE AUTHOR

Anuj Mahajan

A Multifaceted Life Coach, Entrepreneur, and Visionary

Anuj Mahajan is a true Renaissance man—a multifaceted individual who has carved his path through various domains, leaving a lasting impact on each one. His journey is a testament to the power of resilience, personal growth, and the pursuit of one's passions.

Entrepreneurship and Leadership

Anuj's entrepreneurial spirit was evident from an early age. His foray into the world of business began with Vestige Marketing Pvt Ltd, where he achieved the prestigious title of Crown Director. Vestige, known as India's No. 1 direct selling company, recognized Anuj's exceptional leadership and entrepreneurial prowess. Through his dedication and strategic thinking, Anuj has played a pivotal role in the growth and success of Vestige.

Media Maestro

Anuj Mahajan is not just an entrepreneur but also a media maestro. With over 30 years of experience in the media industry, Anuj has a profound understanding of the power of communication and storytelling. As the Managing Director of Nuteq Entertainment, he has been at the forefront of producing content that captivates audiences across various platforms.

Coach Extraordinaire

Anuj's journey took a transformative turn when he embraced the role of a life coach. He is a certified coach with the Indian Coach Federation (ICF), specializing in career transitions, business coaching, and life coaching. His expertise in Neuro-Linguistic Programming (NLP) adds depth to his coaching abilities, allowing him to guide individuals toward personal and professional breakthroughs.

Motivational Speaker and Educator

Anuj Mahajan is more than just a coach; he is a motivational force to be reckoned with. His captivating speeches and training sessions have inspired thousands worldwide. With over 13 years of experience as an international motivational speaker and network marketing expert, Anuj brings real-world experiences and wisdom to his audiences.

Passion for Social Impact

While Anuj excels in the realms of entrepreneurship, coaching, and media, his heart is deeply committed to social impact. He firmly believes that individuals have the power to change the world, and he dedicates his time and efforts to contribute meaningfully to people's lives. Through his social initiatives and leadership roles, Anuj strives to make a positive difference in the communities he touches.

A Global Reach

Anuj's influence extends far beyond geographical boundaries. He has conducted training events, conferences, and seminars globally, leaving a trail of inspired individuals in his wake. With a passion for personal development, leadership, mindfulness, and cultivating positivity, Anuj has become a sought-after speaker and mentor.

Areas of Expertise

Anuj Mahajan's expertise spans a wide spectrum of domains, reflecting his multifaceted persona:

Executive Coaching: Anuj excels in coaching executives to reach their full potential, guiding them to make impactful decisions and lead with clarity and purpose.

Leadership Development: With a wealth of leadership experience, Anuj empowers individuals and teams to enhance their leadership skills and drive success.

Neuro-Linguistic Programming (NLP): Anuj's proficiency in NLP enables him to help clients overcome mental barriers and achieve personal and professional breakthroughs.

Entrepreneur Development: Anuj's entrepreneurial journey makes him a trusted guide for aspiring entrepreneurs, helping them navigate the complexities of business and achieve financial freedom.

Success Coach: As a success coach, Anuj inspires individuals to set and achieve ambitious goals, unlocking their full potential.

Career Development: Anuj's career transition coaching helps individuals navigate career changes and find fulfillment in their professional lives.

Public Speaking: Anuj's dynamic and engaging speaking style captivates audiences and leaves a lasting impression.

Motivational Speaker: Anuj's motivational talks uplift and inspire individuals to overcome obstacles and pursue their dreams with unwavering determination.

Topics of Discussion

Anuj Mahajan's diverse expertise allows him to speak on a wide range of topics, including:

- **Motivation:** Anuj's motivational speeches instill a sense of purpose and drive in his audience, motivating them to take action and achieve their goals.
- **Vestige & Direct Selling Tips:** As a leader in Vestige Marketing Pvt Ltd, Anuj shares valuable insights and tips for success in the direct selling industry.
- **Career Transition:** Anuj guides individuals through the process of transitioning to new careers, helping them find fulfillment and success in their chosen paths.
- **Destress:** Stress management is a critical aspect of well-being, and Anuj offers strategies to help individuals destress and achieve a balanced life.
- **Work-Life Balance:** Achieving a harmonious balance between work and personal life is crucial for overall happiness, and Anuj provides practical advice on this topic.

- **Mindfulness:** Anuj's deep understanding of mindfulness practices allows him to help individuals cultivate presence, reduce stress, and enhance their overall quality of life.
- **Cultivating Positivity:** Anuj shares insights on fostering a positive mindset and attitude, which can lead to greater success and happiness.

In a world where specialization is often celebrated, Anuj Mahajan stands as a testament to the boundless potential of the multifaceted individual. His journey from entrepreneurship to coaching, media, and social impact is an inspiring example of how diverse passions and expertise can come together to create a life of purpose, influence, and fulfillment. As an educator, mentor, and motivational force, Anuj continues to make a profound impact on the lives of many, guiding them toward personal and professional excellence.

ENDNOTES

This eBook, "On-the-Go Mindfulness: Simple Practices for Busy Professionals," has been crafted from a rich tapestry of experiences and wisdom accumulated over 30 years of media expertise and certification as a business coach.

It represents a sincere endeavor to share valuable insights and practical mindfulness techniques to enhance the lives of busy professionals. We hope that the knowledge and guidance within these pages inspire mindfulness and bring about positive transformations in your personal and professional journey.

Thank you for embarking on this mindfulness adventure with us.

Printed in Great Britain
by Amazon

29868101R00040